PETER BENNETT

Healing Your Back Naturally

Practical Tips for Low Back Pain Relief

Contents

1

Disclaimer

The information provided in this book is intended for general informational purposes only and is not a substitute for professional medical advice, diagnosis, or treatment. Always seek the advice of a qualified healthcare professional regarding any medical condition or before starting any exercise program.

While the author, Dr. Peter Bennett, is a chiropractor and health coach with over 20 years of experience, the content of this book is not meant to replace personalised medical guidance. Each individual's situation is unique, and the information provided may not be suitable for everyone. The author and publisher disclaim any liability for any adverse effects resulting from the use or application of the information presented in this book.

Furthermore, it is important to recognise that the field of medicine is constantly evolving, and new research may emerge that could change or challenge the information provided in this book. Therefore, readers are encouraged to stay informed and consult with healthcare professionals for the most up-to-date and accurate information regarding their specific health concerns.

Readers should use their discretion and consult with a qualified healthcare professional before implementing any recommendations, exercises, or strategies discussed in this book, especially if they have pre-existing medical conditions, are pregnant, or have any concerns about their health. Individual results may vary, and it is important to listen to your body and adjust any exercises or treatments according to your own comfort and abilities.

In conclusion, this book is intended to provide general information and guidance for managing low back pain. It is not a substitute for professional medical advice, diagnosis, or treatment. Readers should consult with qualified healthcare professionals for personalised advice and care. The author and publisher disclaim any responsibility for any loss or risk resulting from the use or misuse of the information presented in this book.

2

Introduction

Welcome to "Healing Your Back Naturally: Practical Tips for Low Back Pain Relief"! In this book, we'll embark on a journey to understand low back pain and explore holistic, gentle approaches to alleviate it. I'm Dr. Peter Bennett, a chiropractor and health coach with over 20 years of experience, and I'm thrilled to share my knowledge and insights with you.

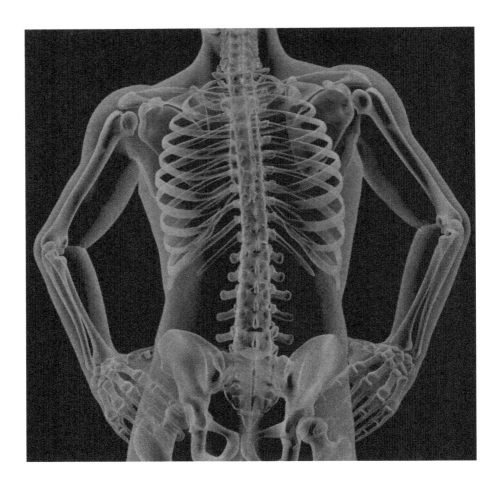

Low back pain has become a prevalent issue in our modern society, affecting people of all ages and backgrounds. It can be debilitating, limiting our ability to perform everyday tasks and enjoy life to the fullest. But the good news is that there are practical steps we can take to find relief and restore balance to our backs.

In our quest for pain relief, it's essential to adopt a holistic approach. Holistic means considering the whole person—body, mind, and spirit—rather than just focusing on the symptoms. Our bodies are intricate systems, and when one part is out of balance, it can impact other areas as well. By addressing the underlying causes of low back pain and nurturing our overall well-being, we can achieve long-lasting relief and promote optimal health.

In the following chapters, we will explore various aspects of low back pain and offer easy-to-implement strategies for relief. We'll start by delving into the fundamentals, helping you gain a deeper understanding of what causes low back pain in the first place. By unraveling the mysteries behind the discomfort, we can empower ourselves to make informed choices and take positive action.

Creating a supportive environment is a crucial step in finding relief. We spend a significant portion of our time sitting, whether at work or home, and improper ergonomics can worsen back pain. Throughout this book, you'll discover practical tips for designing an ergonomic workspace and learn how to optimize your sleep posture to minimise strain on your back. We'll also explore how to arrange your living environment to promote back-friendly habits.

Movement is key to maintaining a healthy back, but it's essential to approach it with care and gentleness. In the chapters ahead, we'll explore a range of gentle exercises and stretches that can improve flexibility, strengthen core muscles, and alleviate low back pain. I'll guide you through each exercise, emphasizing proper form and the importance of listening to your body's signals. Remember, the goal is to build strength and flexibility gradually, not to push yourself beyond your limits.

Beyond physical movement, we'll delve into the realm of mind-body techniques for pain relief. Our mental and emotional well-being play a significant role in how we experience and manage pain. By incorporating mindfulness meditation, relaxation exercises, and stress reduction techniques into our daily routine, we can cultivate a calm and resilient state of mind that supports our overall well-being.

What we put into our bodies matters, too. Nutrition and lifestyle choices can either contribute to or alleviate inflammation, a common culprit in low back pain. In this book, we'll explore the role of anti-inflammatory foods and supplements, as well as the impact of maintaining a healthy weight on our backs. Small changes in our dietary habits can have a profound effect on our pain levels and overall health.

Posture and body mechanics are often overlooked aspects of back health, but they can make a world of difference. By maintaining proper posture and practicing good body mechanics during daily activities, such as lifting, bending, and reaching, we can reduce strain on our backs and prevent further discomfort. I'll provide practical tips and guidance to help you incorporate better posture and body mechanics into your everyday life.

Throughout this book, I encourage you to create a sustainable plan that incorporates the tips and strategies that resonate with you. Self-care is a journey, and finding what works best for your body and lifestyle is key. Keep track of your progress, set realistic goals, and remember to be patient and kind to yourself along the way.

Are you ready to take control of your low back pain and embark on a path towards relief and well-being? Let's dive into the practical tips and strategies that will bring your back back in balance. Together, we'll unlock the secrets to a pain-free life and rediscover the joy of living without limitations.

3

When to Seek Emergency Medical Treatment for Low Back Pain

When it comes to low back pain, most cases can be managed with conservative measures and self-care. However, there are certain situations where seeking emergency medical treatment is necessary. It's important to be aware of the signs and symptoms that warrant immediate attention to ensure your safety and well-being. In this chapter, we will discuss when you should seek emergency medical treatment for low back pain.

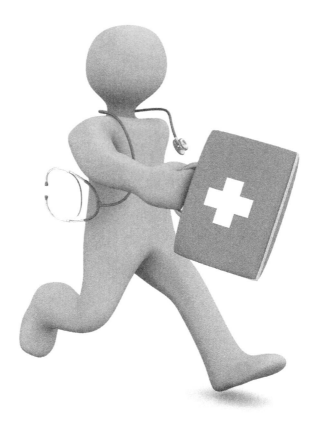

Red Flags and Warning Signs

Low back pain can sometimes be a symptom of a more serious underlying condition. Here are some red flags and warning signs that indicate the need for immediate medical attention:

1. Severe and Sudden Onset: If your low back pain is sudden, severe, and unrelenting, it could be a sign of a serious condition, such as a spinal fracture or ruptured disc.

2. Numbness or Weakness: If you experience sudden numbness or weakness in the legs or difficulty controlling your bladder or bowel movements, it may indicate a condition called cauda equina syndrome. This is a medical emergency that requires immediate attention.

3. Trauma or Injury: If your low back pain is the result of a fall, car accident, or any significant trauma, it's important to seek medical attention. Trauma can lead to fractures or other spinal injuries that require immediate evaluation and treatment.

4. Loss of Bladder or Bowel Control: If you experience a loss of bladder or bowel control along with low back pain, it may indicate a serious condition affecting the nerves in the lower spine. This requires urgent medical attention.

Persistent or Worsening Symptoms

Persistent or worsening symptoms may indicate an underlying problem. It's important to seek medical attention if you experience:

1. Unrelenting Pain: If your low back pain persists or worsens despite conservative measures, it may indicate a more significant issue that requires medical evaluation.

2. Pain Radiating Down the Leg: If your pain radiates down the leg, especially below the knee, it may be a sign of nerve compression or irritation, such as a herniated disc or spinal stenosis. Prompt medical evaluation is necessary in such cases.

3. Fever and Infection Signs: If you have low back pain accompanied by a fever, chills, or signs of infection such as redness, warmth, or swelling, it may indicate an infection in the spine. Infections require immediate medical attention to prevent further complications.

When in Doubt, Seek Advice

It's always better to err on the side of caution when it comes to your health. If you're unsure whether your low back pain requires emergency medical treatment, it's best to seek medical advice. Consulting with a healthcare professional can help determine the appropriate course of action based on your specific symptoms and medical history.

Don't Delay Emergency Treatment

If you experience any of the red flags or warning signs mentioned earlier, it's crucial not to delay seeking emergency medical treatment. Time is of the essence when it comes to certain conditions, and prompt evaluation and treatment can prevent further complications and improve outcomes.

Conclusion:

While most cases of low back pain can be managed with conservative measures, there are instances where seeking emergency medical treatment is necessary. It's important to recognise the red flags and warning signs that warrant immediate attention. If you experience severe and sudden onset of pain, numbness or weakness in the legs, trauma or injury, loss of bladder or bowel control, persistent or worsening symptoms, or signs of infection, it's crucial to seek medical advice without delay. Your health and well-being should always be a top priority, and seeking timely medical attention ensures that you receive the necessary care and treatment for your low back pain.

4

Medication for Low Back Pain

As a chiropractor, my expertise lies in holistic approaches to managing low back pain, focusing on natural therapies, lifestyle modifications, and non-invasive treatments. While these approaches can be effective for many individuals, there are instances where medication may be necessary to provide relief. However, it's important to note that I am not a medical doctor, and medication should always be prescribed and supervised by a qualified healthcare professional. In this chapter, we will explore the role of medication in managing low back pain and emphasize the importance of seeking medical advice.

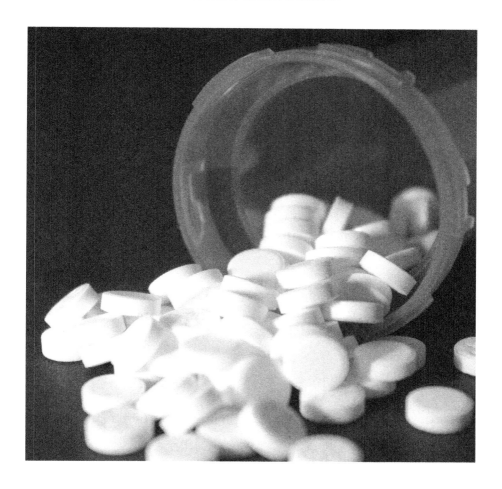

The Role of Medication in Low Back Pain Management

Medication can play a significant role in managing low back pain, particularly in cases where conservative measures alone may not provide sufficient relief. Here are some common types of medications used for low back pain:

1. Over-the-Counter (OTC) Pain Relievers:

Non-prescription pain relievers such as acetaminophen (paracetemol) or non steroidal anti-inflammatory drugs (NSAIDs) like ibuprofen or naproxen can help reduce pain and inflammation associated with low back pain.

2. Muscle Relaxants:

Muscle relaxants may be prescribed to alleviate muscle spasms and promote relaxation in the back muscles. They can provide short-term relief, but they may cause drowsiness and other side effects.

3. Prescription Pain Medications:

In severe cases, stronger pain medications such as opioids may be prescribed for short-term use to manage severe pain. However, due to their potential for addiction and side effects, they should be used with caution and under the supervision of a healthcare professional.

4. Nerve Pain Medications:

Certain medications, such as gabapentin or pregabalin, may be prescribed to help manage nerve-related pain, such as that caused by a herniated disc or nerve compression.

Seeking Medical Advice for Medication

While medication can provide temporary relief for low back pain, it is essential to seek medical advice before initiating any medication regimen. Here's why it's important to consult with a qualified healthcare professional:

1. Accurate Diagnosis:

A healthcare professional will assess your condition, perform a thorough evaluation, and provide an accurate diagnosis. This ensures that the appropriate medication is prescribed based on the underlying cause of your low back pain.

2. Personalised Treatment Plan:

A healthcare professional will tailor a treatment plan to your specific needs, taking into account your medical history, existing conditions, and potential drug interactions. They will determine the most suitable medication and dosage for your situation.

3. Monitoring and Safety:

A healthcare professional will monitor your response to medication, adjust dosages as needed, and ensure your safety throughout the treatment process. They can also address any concerns or side effects that may arise.

4. Holistic Approach:

Seeking medical advice allows for a comprehensive approach to low back pain management. A healthcare professional can recommend a combination of medication, physical therapy, lifestyle modifications, and other appropriate treatments for optimal outcomes.

Integrating Medication with Holistic Approaches

While medication may be part of your low back pain management plan, it's important to remember that it should be integrated with holistic approaches and lifestyle modifications. These include exercise, stretching, proper ergonomics, stress reduction techniques, and maintaining a healthy weight. Holistic approaches work in synergy with medication to support long-term pain relief and overall well-being.

Conclusion:

Medication can be a valuable tool in managing low back pain, but it should always be prescribed and supervised by a qualified healthcare professional. As a chiropractor, my focus is on holistic approaches and non-invasive treatments. However, I recognise the importance of seeking medical advice when medication is necessary. Consult with a healthcare professional to receive an accurate diagnosis, personalised treatment plan, and ongoing monitoring. Remember to integrate medication with holistic approaches and lifestyle modifications for the most comprehensive and effective management of your low back pain.

5

The Dangers of Blocking Pain Signals

Pain is a natural and essential response that alerts us to potential harm or injury. While it may be tempting to block pain signals when experiencing low back pain, it is important to understand the potential dangers associated with this approach. In this section, we will explore the risks and limitations of blocking pain signals and why it is crucial to address the underlying causes of low back pain.

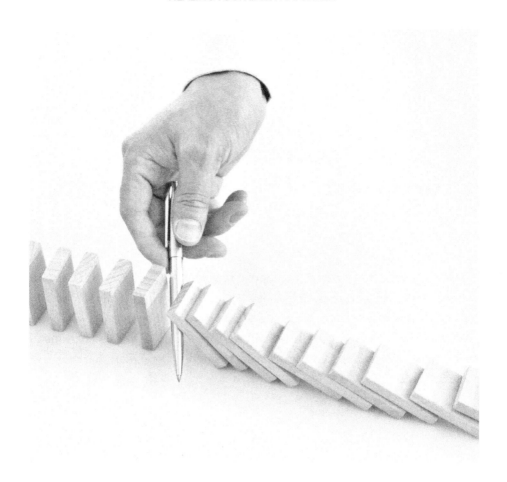

1. Masking Underlying Issues:

Pain serves as a warning sign, signaling that something is wrong in the body. By blocking pain signals without addressing the root cause, we may mask underlying issues that require attention. It is essential to identify and treat the source of pain to prevent further damage or complications.

2. Delayed Healing:

Pain acts as a protective mechanism, limiting our movements and activities to allow the body to heal. By blocking pain signals, we may inadvertently push ourselves beyond our limits, potentially aggravating the underlying condition and hindering the healing process. Delayed healing can lead to chronic pain and long-term complications.

3. Increased Risk of Further Injury:

Pain acts as a natural mechanism that prevents us from engaging in activities that may further injure the affected area. By blocking pain signals, we may engage in movements or behaviors that put us at risk of exacerbating the existing injury or developing new ones. This can lead to more severe and long-lasting consequences.

4. Dependency on Medications:

Blocking pain signals through medications can create a reliance on these drugs for pain management. Long-term use of certain pain medications, such as opioids, can lead to dependency, addiction, and associated health risks. It is important to explore alternative strategies and address the underlying causes of pain to minimise reliance on medications.

5. Lack of Diagnostic Clarity:

Pain serves as a valuable diagnostic tool, helping healthcare professionals identify the source and nature of the problem. By blocking pain signals, we may make it more challenging for professionals to accurately diagnose the underlying condition, potentially delaying appropriate treatment and prolonging the recovery process.

6. Psychological and Emotional Impact:

Pain is not solely a physical sensation but can also impact our psychological and emotional well-being. By blocking pain signals without addressing the underlying causes, we may neglect the psychological and emotional aspects associated with chronic pain, such as anxiety, depression, and decreased quality of life. It is essential to take a holistic approach that addresses both the physical and emotional aspects of low back pain.

Conclusion:

While it may be tempting to block pain signals when experiencing low back pain, it is important to consider the potential dangers and limitations of this approach. Pain serves as a protective mechanism, signaling underlying issues and allowing the body to heal. By addressing the root causes of low back pain and seeking appropriate treatment, we can promote healing, reduce the risk of further injury, and minimise the need for pain-blocking medications. Taking a holistic approach that encompasses physical, psychological, and emotional well-being is key to effectively managing low back pain and achieving long-term relief.

6

Spinal Health and Low Back Pain

The spine is a remarkable structure that provides support, stability, and mobility to our bodies. It consists of a series of bones called vertebrae, which are stacked on top of each other, forming the spinal column. Understanding the intricate relationship between the spine and low back pain is crucial for managing and preventing discomfort. In this chapter, we will explore the key elements of the spine and how they relate to low back pain.

The Structure of the Spine

The spine is divided into several regions, including the cervical (neck), thoracic (upper back), lumbar (lower back), sacrum, and coccyx (tailbone). The lumbar region, specifically, is where low back pain commonly originates. The vertebrae in the lumbar spine are larger and more flexible to support movement and absorb forces.

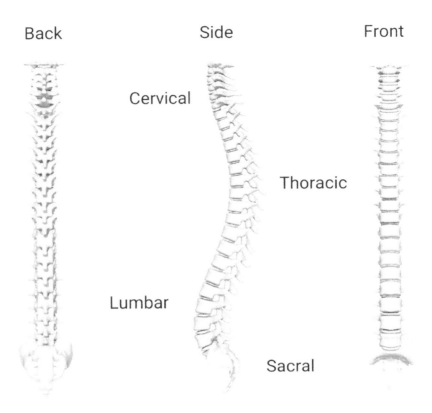

Each vertebra has bony projections called spinous processes and transverse processes, which provide attachment points for muscles and ligaments. Between each pair of vertebrae are intervertebral discs, composed of a gel-like center (nucleus pulposus) surrounded by a tough outer ring (annulus fibrosus). These discs act as shock absorbers and facilitate spinal flexibility.

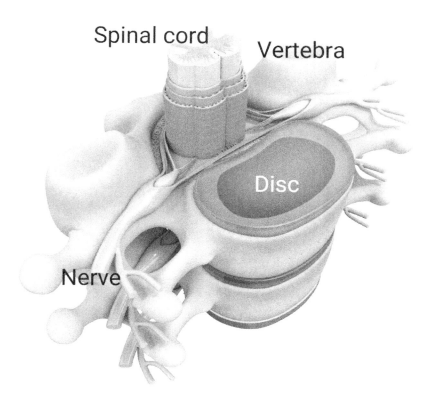

Spinal Alignment and Posture

Proper spinal alignment and posture are essential for maintaining a healthy back and preventing low back pain. When the spine is properly aligned, it distributes forces evenly, reducing stress on individual structures. Poor posture, on the other hand, can place excessive strain on the low back, leading to pain and discomfort.

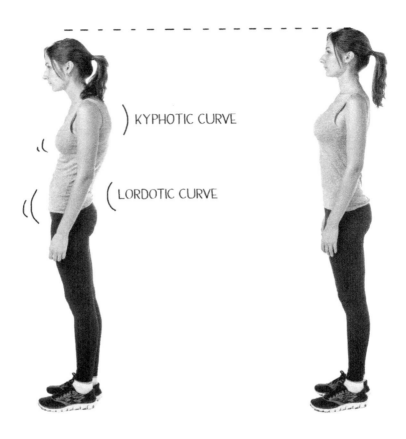

KYPHOTIC CURVE

LORDOTIC CURVE

Maintaining good posture involves aligning the ears, shoulders, hips, and ankles in a straight line. This alignment helps the natural curves of the spine (lordosis in the neck and low back, and kyphosis in the upper back) remain balanced. Engaging in exercises that strengthen the core muscles and practicing proper body mechanics during daily activities further support optimal spinal alignment.

Common Spinal Conditions that Contribute to Low Back Pain

Several spinal conditions can contribute to low back pain. Understanding these conditions can help identify potential sources of discomfort and guide appropriate treatment approaches. Here are a few common conditions:

1. Muscle Strain:

Strained or overworked muscles in the low back can cause pain and stiffness. This can result from poor lifting techniques, sudden movements, or prolonged sitting or standing in an improper posture.

2. Herniated Disc:

When the outer ring of an intervertebral disc weakens or tears, the gel-like center can protrude, irritating nearby nerves. This can lead to localized pain, as well as pain, numbness, or tingling radiating down the leg, known as sciatica.

3. Spinal Stenosis:

Spinal stenosis refers to the narrowing of the spinal canal, which can compress the spinal cord and nerves. This can result in low back pain, as well as symptoms like leg weakness, numbness, or difficulty with walking.

4. Degenerative Disc Disease:

As we age, the intervertebral discs gradually lose moisture and height, causing them to become less effective as shock absorbers. This can lead to low back pain and stiffness.

The Importance of Spinal Health for Low Back Pain Prevention

Maintaining a healthy spine is key to preventing low back pain. Here are some essential practices to promote spinal health:

1. Exercise Regularly:

Engage in exercises that strengthen the core muscles, improve flexibility, and promote proper spinal alignment. This includes activities like yoga, Pilates, and strength training.

2. Practice Good Posture:

Be mindful of your posture throughout the day, whether sitting, standing, or walking. Avoid slouching or excessive rounding of the low back.

3. Lift Properly:

When lifting objects, use your legs and not your back to avoid straining the low back. Bend at the knees, keep the object close to your body, and engage your core muscles.

4. Maintain a Healthy Weight:

Excess weight places added stress on the spine, increasing the risk of low back pain. Maintaining a healthy weight through proper nutrition and regular exercise can alleviate strain on the low back.

Conclusion:

The spine plays a vital role in low back pain, as it provides support, stability, and mobility to our bodies. Understanding the structure and function of the spine helps us recognise how posture, spinal alignment, and common spinal conditions can contribute to low back pain. By practicing good posture, engaging in regular exercise, lifting properly, and maintaining a healthy weight, we can promote spinal health and reduce the risk of low back pain. Taking care of our spines is essential for leading a pain-free and active life.

7

The Importance of Regular Spinal Health Checks

"There once was a spine, straight and true,
Supporting us in all that we do.
With discs in between,
It keeps us serene,
Oh, spine, we're grateful for you!"
Peter Bennett

Maintaining good spinal health is crucial for overall well-being and quality of life. Your spine serves as the central pillar of support for your body, protecting the delicate spinal cord and ensuring proper nerve function. While it's easy to take your spine for granted, regular spinal health checks are essential for early detection and prevention of potential issues. In this chapter, we will explore the importance of getting your spinal health checked regularly and how it can positively impact your overall health.

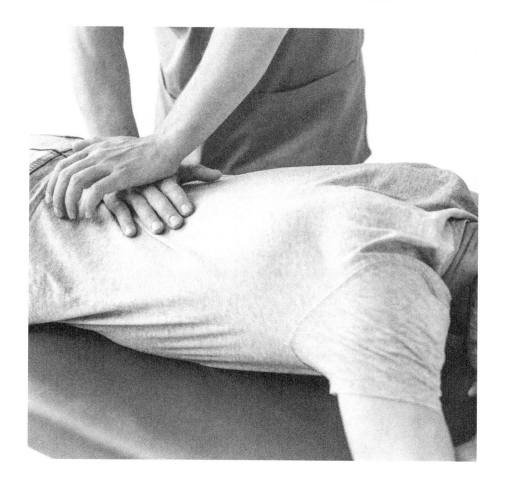

Early Detection of Spinal Issues

Regular spinal health checks allow spinal therapists to assess the condition of your spine and identify any potential issues before they become major concerns. Just like regular dental check-ups or annual physical exams, spinal health checks provide an opportunity to catch problems in their early stages when they are more manageable and less likely to cause significant discomfort or limitations.

1. Identifying Misalignments:

Misalignments in the spine, known as subluxations, can occur due to poor posture, repetitive movements, injuries, or other factors. Regular spinal health checks can help detect and correct these misalignments, allowing for optimal spinal function and reducing the risk of pain or nerve interference.

2. Addressing Spinal Degeneration:

Over time, the spine can undergo degenerative changes, such as disc degeneration or arthritis. Regular spinal health checks enable spinal therapists to monitor these changes and implement appropriate interventions to slow down the progression and minimize their impact on your health.

3. Assessing Nerve Function:

The spinal cord and nerves travel through the spine, connecting the brain to the rest of the body. Any disruption or interference in nerve function can lead to pain, dysfunction, or other health issues. Regular spinal health checks help assess nerve function and detect any potential areas of concern.

Damage Prevention and Maintenance of Spinal Health

Regular spinal health checks are not just about addressing existing issues; they also play a vital role in preventing future problems and maintaining optimal spinal health. Through preventative care and maintenance, you can proactively support the long-term health and function of your spine.

1. Maintaining Proper Alignment:

Regular spinal health checks help ensure that your spine maintains proper alignment, reducing the risk of subluxations and associated issues. By addressing misalignments early on, spinal therapists can provide appropriate adjustments or therapies to realign the spine and restore optimal function.

2. Promoting Spinal Flexibility:

As we age, the spine naturally loses some of its flexibility. Regular spinal health checks allow spinal therapists to assess your spinal flexibility and provide recommendations for exercises, stretches, or therapies to improve and maintain mobility.

3. Managing Everyday Stressors:

Daily activities, such as sitting for extended periods, poor posture, or repetitive movements, can place stress on the spine. Regular spinal health checks enable spinal therapists to assess how these stressors may be affecting your spine and offer guidance on lifestyle modifications, ergonomics, and exercises to minimize their impact.

Holistic Health Benefits

Beyond the specific benefits to your spine, regular spinal health checks offer holistic health benefits that extend to other areas of your well-being. A healthy spine is linked to improved overall health and vitality.

1. Enhanced Nervous System Function:

Your spine houses the spinal cord, which serves as a communication pathway between your brain and body. A properly functioning spine ensures optimal nerve flow and communication, supporting overall bodily function and well-being.

2. Improved Posture and Balance:

Regular spinal health checks can help correct postural imbalances and improve spinal alignment. This, in turn, promotes better posture, balance, and body mechanics, reducing the risk of injuries and enhancing overall physical performance.

3. Better Energy and Vitality:

When your spine is properly aligned and your nervous system is functioning optimally, your body can operate at its best. This can result in increased energy levels, improved sleep quality, and a greater sense of vitality and well-being.

Conclusion:

Regular spinal health checks are an essential component of maintaining overall health and well-being. By addressing spinal issues in their early stages, preventing future problems, and promoting optimal spinal function, you can support your long-term spinal health and enjoy a better quality of life. Remember to seek qualified spinal therapists specializing in spinal care and prioritise regular check-ups to reap the benefits of a healthy spine for years to come.

8

Creating a Back Safe Environment

Ergonomic Workspaces for Back Health

Creating an ergonomic workspace is essential for reducing strain on the back and promoting a pain-free work experience. Here are some tips to help you optimize your workspace:

1. Chair and Desk:

Choose an adjustable chair that provides proper lumbar support and promotes good posture. Your feet should be flat on the floor, and your knees should be at a 90-degree angle. Pair it with a desk at the appropriate height to ensure your arms are parallel to the desk surface.

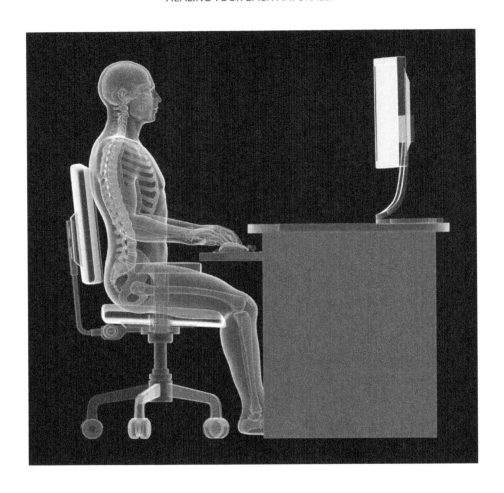

2. Monitor Placement:

Position your computer monitor at eye level to avoid straining your neck and upper back. Use a monitor stand or adjust the height of your monitor accordingly.

3. Keyboard and Mouse:

Use an ergonomic keyboard and mouse that allow your hands and wrists to maintain a neutral position. This can help prevent strain and discomfort in the wrists, arms, and shoulders.

4. Breaks and Movement:

Take frequent breaks to stretch and move around. Sitting for prolonged periods can contribute to back pain. Incorporate exercises and stretches that target the back, neck, and shoulders to alleviate tension.

Sleep Posture and Mattress Selection

Proper sleep posture and mattress selection play a crucial role in maintaining a healthy back. Follow these guidelines for better sleep and back support:

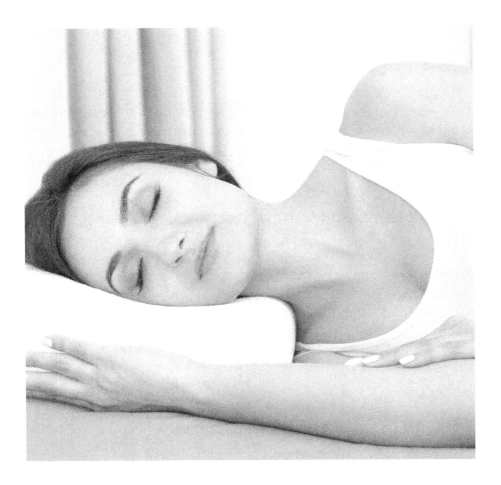

1. Mattress Firmness:

Choose a mattress that provides adequate support for your back. A medium-firm mattress is generally recommended, as it offers a balance between comfort and support. Avoid overly soft or sagging mattresses, as they may cause spinal misalignment and worsen back pain.

2. Pillow Support:

Use a pillow that supports the natural curve of your neck and keeps your spine aligned while you sleep. Consider using a contoured cervical pillow or one that adjusts to your preferred sleeping position.

3. Sleep Position:

Sleeping on your back or side is generally better for back health than sleeping on your stomach. If you sleep on your back, place a pillow under your knees to maintain a neutral spine. If you sleep on your side, tuck a pillow between your knees for added support.

4. Mattress Maintenance:

Rotate and flip your mattress regularly to prevent uneven wear and maintain its supportive properties. This can help prolong the lifespan of your mattress and ensure consistent back support.

Back-Friendly Home Environment

Creating a back-friendly home environment involves arranging furniture and incorporating accessories that promote good posture and reduce strain. Consider the following tips:

1. Sitting Areas:

Choose chairs and sofas with proper lumbar support and ensure they are at the right height to maintain good posture. Add cushions or lumbar rolls to provide additional support if needed.

2. Standing Workstations:

Consider incorporating a standing desk or adjustable desk converter into your home office. Alternate between sitting and standing throughout the day to reduce the strain on your back and promote better blood circulation.

3. Lifting and Carrying:

Practice proper body mechanics when lifting and carrying objects. Bend your knees, keep your back straight, and engage your core muscles. Use assistive devices like trolleys or carts for heavier items whenever possible.

4. Back-Friendly Accessories:

Incorporate back-friendly accessories throughout your home. Use supportive pillows and cushions while sitting or relaxing. Invest in a comfortable and supportive chair for activities such as reading or watching television.

Conclusion:

Creating a supportive environment is crucial for maintaining a healthy back and preventing low back pain. By implementing ergonomic principles in your workspace, optimizing your sleep posture and mattress selection, and arranging your home with back-friendly furniture and accessories, you can significantly reduce strain on your back and promote better spinal alignment. Remember, small changes can make a big difference in your overall comfort and well-being.

9

Tips for Safe Lifting and Handling

Lifting and handling objects is a common part of our daily lives, but it can also be a significant source of low back pain and injury if not done properly. Whether you're moving furniture, carrying groceries, or lifting weights at the gym, it's essential to prioritise your safety and protect your low back. In this chapter, we will explore practical tips for safe lifting and handling to prevent low back pain and reduce the risk of injury.

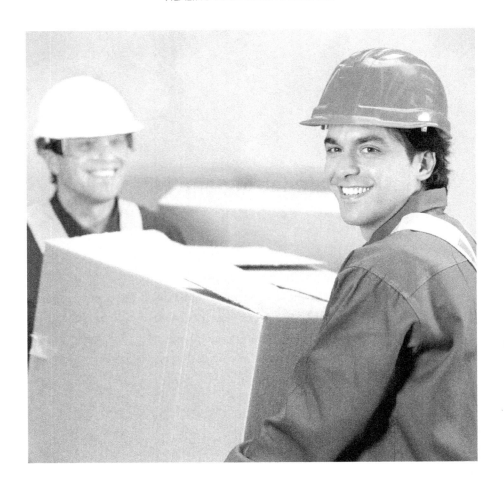

Preparing for the Lift

Proper preparation is crucial to ensure a safe lifting experience. Consider the following tips before attempting to lift or handle an object:

1. Assess the Load:

Before lifting, evaluate the weight and size of the object. If it seems too heavy or awkward to handle alone, seek assistance or use appropriate equipment like dollies or hand trucks.

2. Clear the Path:

Ensure the pathway is clear of any obstacles, debris, or tripping hazards. Creating a clear path allows you to focus on the lift without the risk of accidents or sudden disruptions.

3. Warm Up:

Before engaging in any heavy lifting, warm up your muscles and joints with light cardiovascular exercise and dynamic stretching. This helps increase blood flow and prepares your body for the physical demands of lifting.

Proper Lifting Technique

Using proper lifting technique is essential to protect your low back from strain and injury. Follow these guidelines when lifting and handling objects:

1. Maintain Good Posture:

Stand with your feet shoulder-width apart, toes pointing forward. Keep your back straight, shoulders back, and your head aligned with your spine. Avoid slouching or rounding your low back during the lift.

2. Bend Your Knees:

To initiate the lift, squat down by bending your knees, not your back. Keep your heels on the ground and your back straight as you lower yourself to the level of the object.

3. Get a Firm Grip:

Ensure you have a secure and firm grip on the object before attempting to lift. Use both hands and avoid gripping with just your fingers or fingertips.

4. Lift with Your Legs:

Engage your leg muscles, particularly your quadriceps and glutes, as you begin to lift. Push through your heels and straighten your legs, using the power of your legs instead of your back to lift the object.

5. Keep the Load Close:

Keep the object as close to your body as possible while lifting. This reduces the strain on your low back and provides better control over the weight.

Additional Tips for Safe Handling

In addition to proper lifting technique, there are other tips to ensure safe handling of objects:

1. Avoid Twisting:

When lifting or carrying an object, avoid twisting your body. Instead, pivot your feet and turn your entire body to change direction. Twisting while carrying a heavy load can strain your low back and increase the risk of injury.

2. Pace Yourself:

Take breaks if needed, especially when engaging in prolonged or repetitive lifting tasks. Overexertion can lead to fatigue and decreased lifting technique, increasing the risk of injury.

3. Use Assistive Devices:

If available, use mechanical aids or assistive devices such as dollies, carts, or pulleys to help with heavy or bulky loads. These tools can significantly reduce the strain on your low back.

4. Communicate and Seek Help:

If the object is too heavy or bulky to handle on your own, don't hesitate to ask for assistance. Communicate with others and work together to ensure a safe lifting experience.

Everyday Practices for Low Back Safety

Safe lifting and handling extend beyond specific instances. Incorporate these everyday practices into your routine to promote low back safety:

1. Maintain Fitness and Strength:

Engage in regular exercise and strength-training activities that target your core muscles, including your abdominal and low back muscles. A strong core provides stability and support during lifting and handling tasks.

2. Practice Good Posture:

Maintaining good posture throughout the day, whether sitting, standing, or walking, helps alleviate unnecessary strain on your low back and reduces the risk of injury during lifting activities.

3. Stretch and Rest:

Take regular breaks during prolonged periods of standing, sitting, or repetitive tasks. Incorporate stretching exercises to release tension in your low back and maintain flexibility.

4. Avoid Overloading Bags or Backpacks:

When carrying bags or backpacks, distribute the weight evenly and avoid overloading them. Use both straps for backpacks and consider using bags with wheels for heavier loads.

Conclusion:

Safe lifting and handling practices are essential for protecting your low back and preventing injuries. By preparing properly, using correct lifting technique, and incorporating safe handling practices into your daily routine, you can significantly reduce the risk of low back pain and injury. Remember to prioritise your safety, listen to your body, and seek assistance when necessary. With these tips in mind, you can confidently navigate lifting and handling tasks while maintaining a healthy and pain-free low back.

10

Gentle Exercises to Relieve Low Back Pain

In this chapter, we will explore a variety of gentle exercises that can help alleviate low back pain. These exercises are designed to promote flexibility, strengthen core muscles, and improve overall back health. Remember to consult with a healthcare professional before starting any new exercise regimen, especially if you have underlying health conditions or concerns.

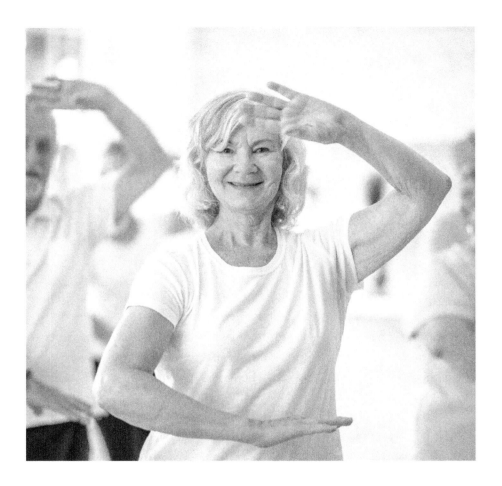

Importance of Gentle Exercises for Low Back Pain Relief

Regular exercise is essential for managing low back pain. Gentle exercises can help improve flexibility, increase strength, and enhance the stability of the core muscles that support the spine. These exercises promote better posture, reduce strain on the back, and alleviate pain. Here are some important benefits of gentle exercises for low back pain relief:

46

1. Improved Flexibility:

Gentle exercises, such as stretching, help improve flexibility in the muscles and soft tissues of the back. Increased flexibility can reduce stiffness, enhance range of motion, and alleviate pain associated with tight muscles.

2. Strengthening Core Muscles:

Weak core muscles can contribute to low back pain. Gentle exercises target the deep abdominal muscles, back extensors, and hip muscles, which provide stability and support to the spine. Strengthening these muscles can reduce the risk of pain and injury.

3. Enhanced Spinal Stability:

Gentle exercises that engage the core muscles help enhance spinal stability. A stable spine is better equipped to withstand the stresses of daily activities and is less prone to strain or injury.

Gentle Exercises for Low Back Pain Relief

When starting any exercise program, it's important to begin slowly and gradually increase intensity and duration. Listen to your body and modify exercises as needed to suit your comfort level. Here are some gentle exercises that can help relieve low back pain:

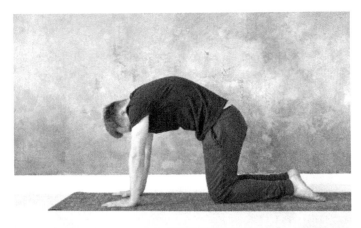

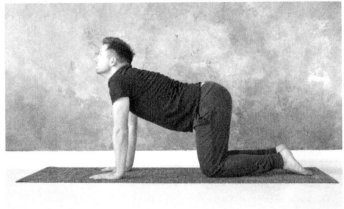

1. Cat-Camel Stretch:

Begin on your hands and knees, with your hands under your shoulders and knees under your hips. Slowly arch your back up towards the ceiling, tucking your chin towards your chest (cat position). Then, gradually lower your belly towards the floor, lifting your head and tailbone upwards (camel position). Repeat this movement in a smooth, flowing motion for several repetitions.

2. Pelvic Tilts:

Lie on your back with your knees bent and feet flat on the floor. Gently tilt your pelvis by flattening your lower back against the floor. Hold for a few seconds, then release. Repeat this movement, focusing on engaging your abdominal muscles.

3. Knee-to-Chest Stretch:

Lie on your back with your knees bent and feet flat on the floor. Slowly bring one knee towards your chest, holding onto the back of your thigh or shin. Hold for 20-30 seconds, then release and repeat with the other leg. This stretch helps release tension in the lower back and stretches the gluteal muscles.

4. Bridge Exercise:

Lie on your back with your knees bent and feet flat on the floor, hip-width apart. Press your feet into the floor as you lift your hips off the ground, creating a straight line from your shoulders to your knees. Hold this position for a few seconds, then lower your hips back down. Repeat for several repetitions, focusing on engaging your glutes and core muscles.

5. Modified Cobra Stretch:

Lie on your stomach with your palms on the floor beside your shoulders. Slowly press your hands into the floor as you lift your chest off the ground, keeping your pelvis and lower body relaxed. Hold for a few seconds, then lower back down. This stretch helps strengthen the back muscles and improves spinal extension.

6. Gentle Yoga or Tai Chi:

Consider incorporating gentle yoga or tai chi classes into your routine. These practices promote flexibility, balance, and relaxation, all of which can contribute to low back pain relief.

Additional Considerations and Tips

Here are some additional considerations and tips to keep in mind when engaging in gentle exercises for low back pain relief:

1. Warm-Up and Cool-Down:

Always warm up before exercising with light cardio activities like brisk walking or cycling. Likewise, cool down with stretches to help prevent muscle soreness and injury.

2. Proper Form:

Pay attention to your posture and form during exercises. Avoid straining or overexerting your back. If an exercise causes pain or discomfort, modify it or consult with a healthcare professional.

3. Gradual Progression:

Start with a few repetitions of each exercise and gradually increase as your body becomes accustomed to the movements. Avoid pushing through pain and give yourself time to adapt and build strength.

4. Variety:

Incorporate a variety of exercises into your routine to target different muscle groups and promote overall back health. This can help prevent muscle imbalances and boredom.

Conclusion:

Gentle exercises can be highly effective in relieving low back pain and promoting overall back health. These exercises improve flexibility, strengthen core muscles, and enhance spinal stability. Remember to consult with a healthcare professional before starting any exercise program and listen to your body's cues. With consistent practice and proper form, gentle exercises can become a valuable tool in managing low back pain and improving your quality of life.

11

Advanced Exercises for a Stronger Low Back

In the previous chapter, we explored various gentle exercises and stretches to alleviate low back pain and promote flexibility. Now, let's take a step further and introduce more advanced exercises that can strengthen your low back muscles, improve stability, and prevent future pain. Additionally, I'm excited to introduce you to my online exercise program, "Beat Back Pain," designed to guide you through these advanced exercises. Let's dive in!

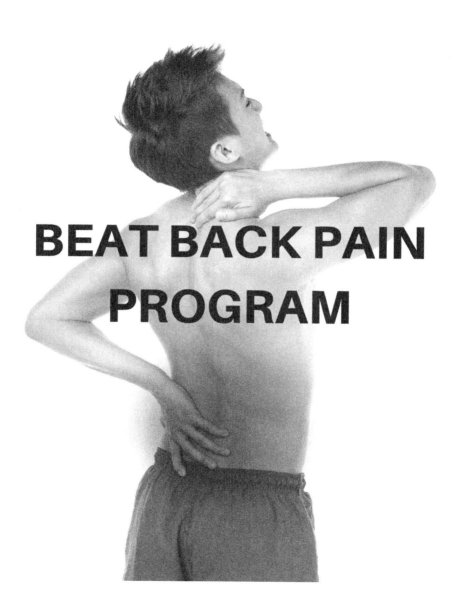

BEAT BACK PAIN PROGRAM

The Importance of Advanced Exercises for Low Back Strength

Building a strong and resilient low back is crucial for maintaining a pain-free and active lifestyle. Advanced exercises target the deep core muscles, including the abdominals, back extensors, and hip muscles. These exercises enhance stability, improve posture, and reduce the risk of future low back pain. It's important to note that before attempting advanced exercises, you should have a solid foundation of core strength and consult with a healthcare professional to ensure they are appropriate for your condition.

Introducing "Beat Back Pain" Online Exercise Program

I'm thrilled to introduce you to "Beat Back Pain," an online exercise program designed to guide you through advanced exercises for low back strength. This program combines my years of experience as a chiropractor and health coach to provide you with a comprehensive and accessible resource for building a stronger low back.

1. Program Overview:

"Beat Back Pain" is a step-by-step program that gradually introduces you to advanced exercises, ensuring proper form and technique. It focuses on strengthening the core muscles, improving flexibility, and promoting overall back health.

2. Guided Video Demonstrations:

The program includes detailed video demonstrations of each exercise, making it easy to follow along and ensure correct execution. You can access the videos at your convenience and review them as needed.

3. Progression and Modifications:

"Beat Back Pain" offers progressive exercises that gradually challenge your low back muscles as you build strength. It also provides modifications for different fitness levels, allowing you to tailor the program to your needs.

4. Warm-up and Cool-down Routines:

The program incorporates warm-up and cool-down routines to prepare your body for exercise and promote proper recovery. These routines help prevent injuries and optimize the benefits of the program.

Sample Advanced Exercises for Low Back Strength

While the complete "Beat Back Pain" program offers a comprehensive set of exercises, here are a few exercises you can do to start with:

1. Plank Variations:

Planks are excellent for strengthening the core, including the low back. "Beat Back Pain" introduces different plank variations, such as side planks, forearm planks, and plank with leg lifts, to challenge and engage your core muscles.

2. Superman:

Lie on your stomach with your arms extended overhead and lift your arms, chest, and legs off the ground simultaneously. Hold for a few seconds, then lower back down. This exercise targets the back extensors and improves spinal stability.

3. Deadlifts:

Using proper form and technique, deadlifts can be an effective exercise for strengthening the low back, glutes, and hamstrings. They improve functional strength and teach proper hip hinge mechanics.

4. Bridging Variations:

Bridges target the glutes and low back muscles. "Beat Back Pain" includes variations such as single-leg bridges or bridges on an unstable surface to challenge stability and increase muscle activation.

Getting Started with "Beat Back Pain"

To get started with the "Beat Back Pain" online exercise program:

1. Visit www.beatbackpain.co.uk to access the program and create an account.

2. Review the program overview and familiarize yourself with the exercises and video demonstrations.

3. Follow the program's progression, starting with the introductory exercises and gradually advancing as you build strength and confidence.

4. Listen to your body, respect your limits, and adjust the program according to your needs. It's important to maintain proper form and technique to prevent injury.

Conclusion:

Building a strong low back is essential for preventing pain and maintaining an active lifestyle. Through advanced exercises, you can strengthen your core muscles, improve stability, and reduce the risk of future low back issues. The "Beat Back Pain" online exercise program offers a comprehensive resource to guide you through these exercises, providing video demonstrations, progression, and modifications. Remember to consult with a healthcare professional to ensure these exercises are suitable for your condition. Get started with "Beat Back Pain" and embark on a journey towards a stronger and pain-free low back.

12

Mind-Body Techniques for Pain Relief

The Power of Mind-Body Connection

The mind-body connection plays a significant role in how we experience and manage pain, including low back pain. By harnessing the power of this connection, we can use various mind-body techniques to alleviate discomfort and promote healing. In this chapter, we will explore some effective techniques that can provide relief from low back pain.

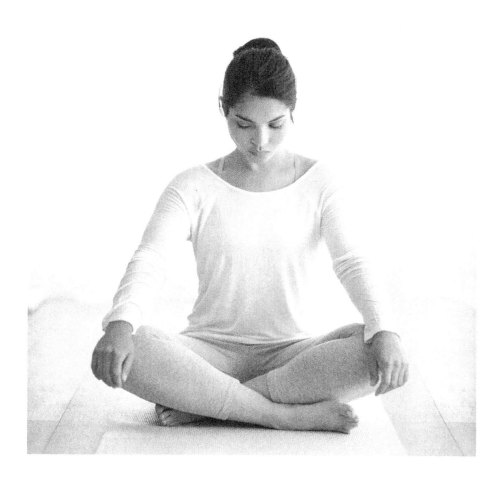

Mindfulness Meditation for Pain Management

Mindfulness meditation is a powerful technique that involves paying attention to the present moment without judgment. It can be particularly beneficial for managing pain, including low back pain. Here's how mindfulness meditation can help:

1. Awareness and Acceptance:

By cultivating awareness of the sensations and thoughts associated with pain, mindfulness meditation allows us to develop a non-judgmental attitude towards our experience. Instead of resisting or fighting the pain, we learn to accept it with compassion and understanding.

2. Pain Distraction:

Mindfulness meditation can act as a helpful distraction from the intensity of low back pain. By shifting our focus to the present moment, we can reduce the perception of pain and develop a sense of calm and relaxation.

3. Stress Reduction:

Mindfulness meditation has been shown to reduce stress levels, which can contribute to the experience of pain. By calming the mind and activating the body's relaxation response, we can alleviate tension in the back and promote pain relief.

Relaxation Techniques for Low Back Pain Relief

Relaxation techniques can be powerful tools for managing low back pain and promoting overall well-being. Here are a few techniques that you can incorporate into your routine:

1. Deep Breathing Exercises:

Deep breathing helps activate the body's relaxation response and reduces stress. Take slow, deep breaths, inhaling deeply through your nose and exhaling fully through your mouth. Focus on the sensation of the breath and allow your body to relax with each exhale.

2. Progressive Muscle Relaxation:

Progressive muscle relaxation involves systematically tensing and relaxing different muscle groups to promote deep relaxation. Starting from your toes and moving up to your head, tense each muscle group for a few seconds, then release the tension, allowing the muscles to relax fully.

3. Guided Imagery:

Guided imagery involves using your imagination to create a calming and soothing mental image. Close your eyes and visualize a peaceful place or engage in a guided imagery meditation that focuses on relaxing the body and mind. This technique can help redirect your attention away from pain and induce a state of deep relaxation.

The Impact of Stress Reduction on Low Back Pain

Stress can have a significant impact on low back pain, as it can worsen muscle tension and increase the perception of pain. By incorporating stress reduction techniques into your daily life, you can alleviate stress and its effects on your back. Here's how stress reduction can help:

1. Relaxation Response:

Engaging in relaxation techniques triggers the body's relaxation response, which counteracts the stress response. This can help reduce muscle tension, lower blood pressure, and promote an overall sense of well-being.

2. Emotional Well-being:

Stress can negatively impact emotional well-being, which in turn affects pain perception. By reducing stress, we can enhance our emotional state and create a positive feedback loop that supports pain relief.

3. Improved Sleep Quality:

Chronic stress can disrupt sleep patterns, leading to increased pain sensitivity and exacerbation of low back pain. By reducing stress and promoting relaxation, we can improve the quality of our sleep, allowing our bodies to heal and regenerate more effectively.

Conclusion:

Mind-body techniques offer powerful tools for managing low back pain and promoting overall well-being. By incorporating mindfulness meditation, relaxation techniques like deep breathing and progressive muscle relaxation, and stress reduction practices, we can effectively reduce pain, promote relaxation, and enhance our emotional well-being. Remember to experiment with different techniques and find the ones that resonate with you the most. Through the mind-body connection, we can harness our inner resources to find relief and regain control over our low back pain.

13

Nutrition and Lifestyle Choices

Understanding the Impact of Diet on Low Back Pain

The food we eat plays a significant role in our overall health, including the management of low back pain. Certain foods can either alleviate or worsen inflammation, which is often associated with low back pain. Understanding the impact of diet on low back pain can empower us to make informed choices that support our well-being.

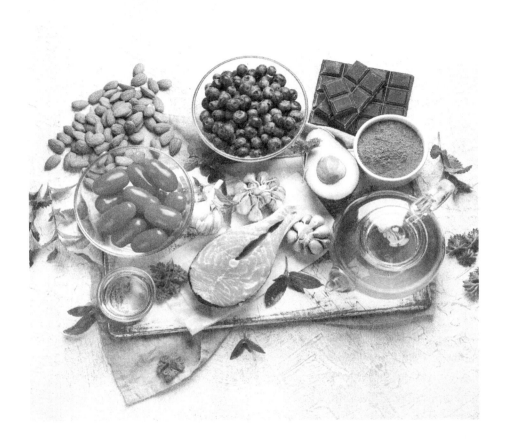

1. Inflammatory Foods:

Some foods, such as processed meats, refined carbohydrates, sugary snacks, and fried foods, can contribute to inflammation in the body. Inflammation can worsen low back pain and prolong the healing process. By reducing our consumption of these foods, we can potentially alleviate inflammation and reduce pain.

2. Anti-Inflammatory Foods:

On the other hand, there are foods that possess anti-inflammatory properties and can help reduce pain and inflammation. Incorporating more of these foods into our diet can provide relief. Examples of anti-inflammatory foods include fatty fish like salmon and sardines, leafy greens, berries, nuts, seeds, olive oil, and turmeric.

Dietary Recommendations for Low Back Pain Relief

Making dietary changes can significantly impact low back pain and overall health. Here are some dietary recommendations to consider:

1. Emphasize Whole Foods:

Focus on a diet rich in whole, unprocessed foods such as fruits, vegetables, whole grains, lean proteins, and healthy fats. These foods provide essential nutrients, antioxidants, and anti-inflammatory compounds that support a healthy back and overall well-being.

2. Omega-3 Fatty Acids:

Increase your intake of omega-3 fatty acids, found in fatty fish, chia seeds, flax seeds, and walnuts. Omega-3 fatty acids have anti-inflammatory properties and can help reduce pain and inflammation in the back.

3. Spices and Herbs:

Incorporate spices and herbs with anti-inflammatory properties into your cooking. Turmeric, ginger, garlic, cinnamon, and rosemary are examples of spices and herbs that can help alleviate inflammation and reduce low back pain.

4. Hydration:

Drink plenty of water to stay hydrated. Proper hydration supports spinal discs and helps maintain their shock-absorbing properties, reducing the risk of back pain.

5. Supplements:

Consider supplements that have been shown to reduce inflammation, such as fish oil or omega-3 supplements, curcumin (the active compound in turmeric), or ginger supplements. However, it's important to consult with a healthcare professional before starting any new supplements.

Weight Management and its Impact on the Back

Maintaining a healthy weight is crucial for managing low back pain. Excess weight puts additional strain on the spine, leading to increased pain and discomfort. Here's how weight management impacts the back:

1. Spinal Load:

Excess weight places a greater load on the spinal structures, including the discs, joints, and muscles. This increased load can lead to accelerated degeneration, disc herniation, and muscle imbalances, exacerbating low back pain.

2. Inflammation and Hormonal Factors:

Adipose tissue (fat) produces inflammatory substances that can contribute to systemic inflammation and pain. Additionally, excess weight can disrupt hormonal balance, further influencing pain perception.

3. Positive Effects of Weight Loss:

Losing excess weight can significantly alleviate low back pain by reducing stress on the spinal structures. Weight loss improves spinal alignment, decreases inflammation, and helps restore proper muscle balance.

4. Healthy Lifestyle:

Weight management is not solely about shedding pounds; it's about adopting a healthy lifestyle. Regular exercise, balanced nutrition, and mindful eating habits contribute to overall well-being, which in turn positively impacts low back pain management.

Conclusion:

Nutrition and lifestyle choices have a profound impact on low back pain management. By reducing inflammation through dietary choices, incorporating anti-inflammatory foods and supplements, and maintaining a healthy weight, we can alleviate pain, support healing, and promote overall back health. Remember to make gradual changes, listen to your body's cues, and consult with a healthcare professional for personalised advice. By nourishing our bodies with the right foods and adopting a healthy lifestyle, we can find relief and thrive with a pain-free back.

14

Posture and Body Mechanics

The Significance of Proper Posture for Low Back Pain

Proper posture is crucial for preventing and relieving low back pain. When we maintain good posture, we distribute the forces and weight-bearing load on our spine more evenly, reducing the strain on the back muscles, discs, and ligaments. Here's why proper posture matters:

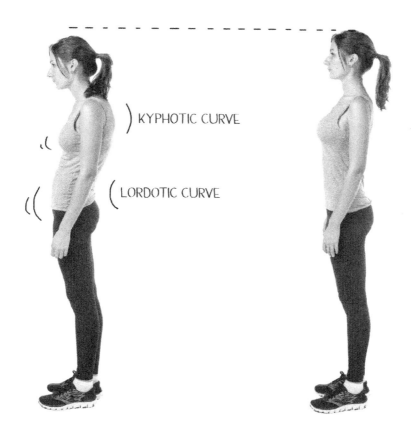

KYPHOTIC CURVE

LORDOTIC CURVE

1. Spinal Alignment:

Good posture helps maintain the natural curves of the spine, including the inward curve of the lower back (lumbar lordosis). When the spine is properly aligned, it can better withstand the stresses of daily activities and minimise the risk of low back pain.

2. Muscle Balance:

Proper posture promotes muscle balance by engaging the core muscles, including the abdominals, back extensors, and hip muscles. These muscles work in harmony to support the spine and prevent excessive strain on the low back.

3. Pressure Distribution:

Maintaining good posture ensures that the weight-bearing load is distributed evenly across the spinal structures. This reduces localized pressure on specific areas, such as the discs, and helps prevent discomfort and pain.

Tips for Maintaining Good Posture

Maintaining good posture throughout the day is essential for preventing low back pain. Here are some practical tips to help you improve and maintain good posture:

1. Sitting Posture:

- Sit with your back against the chair, ensuring that your lower back is supported by the chair's lumbar support or a small cushion.
- Keep your feet flat on the floor or use a footrest if needed.
- Maintain a slight natural curve in your lower back and avoid slouching or leaning forward.
- Position your computer screen at eye level to avoid straining your neck and upper back.

2. Standing Posture:

- Stand tall with your shoulders back and relaxed.
- Engage your core muscles to support your spine and maintain a neutral

pelvis.
- Distribute your weight evenly on both feet, avoiding excessive weight on one side.
- Avoid locking your knees and maintain a slight bend in them.

3. Lifting and Carrying:

- Bend your knees and hinge at your hips when lifting objects from the floor, keeping your back straight.
- Hold the object close to your body and use your leg muscles to lift, avoiding excessive strain on your back.
- Avoid twisting your body while lifting or carrying heavy objects. Instead, pivot your feet to change direction.
- If an object is too heavy or awkward to lift alone, ask for assistance or use lifting aids.

Body Mechanics for Daily Activities

Incorporating proper body mechanics into your daily activities is essential for preventing low back pain. Here are some guidelines for common daily activities:

1. Bending and Reaching:

- Bend your knees and hinge at your hips when bending forward to pick up objects from the ground.
- Avoid rounding your back and use your leg muscles to support the movement.
- When reaching for objects, step closer to them rather than leaning forward

excessively.
- If you need to reach for something overhead, use a stable step stool or ladder to avoid overreaching.

2. Carrying Objects:

- When carrying heavy objects, hold them close to your body and distribute the weight evenly.
- Use both hands whenever possible to balance the load.
- If carrying a bag or backpack, use both shoulder straps to distribute the weight evenly across your back.
- Consider using a backpack or bag with wheels for heavier loads to minimise strain on your back.

3. Sitting and Standing Transitions:

- Avoid sudden movements when transitioning from sitting to standing or vice versa.
- Engage your core muscles and use your leg strength to rise or lower yourself slowly.
- Use a chair with armrests for support when sitting or standing if necessary.

Conclusion:

Maintaining good posture and practicing proper body mechanics are essential for preventing and relieving low back pain. By incorporating these habits into our daily lives, we can reduce strain on the spine, prevent discomfort, and promote a healthy back. Remember to be mindful of your posture while sitting, standing, lifting, and performing daily activities. By making conscious efforts to maintain proper alignment and use proper body mechanics, you can support your back's health and minimise the risk of low back pain.

15

Creating a Sustainable Plan

Developing a Personalised Plan for Low Back Pain Management

Managing low back pain requires a personalised approach that takes into account your unique needs and circumstances. By incorporating the tips and strategies provided throughout this book, you can create a sustainable plan for long-term pain relief. Here's how you can develop your personalised plan:

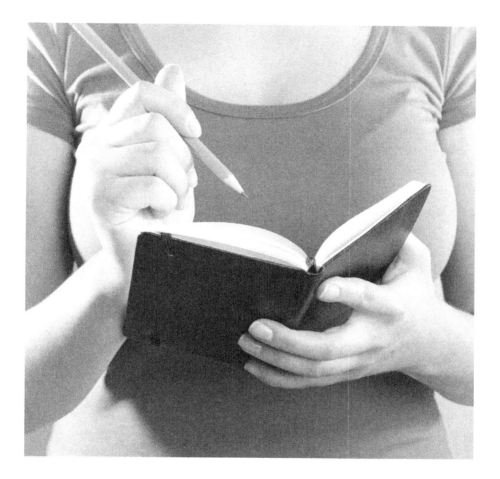

1. Assess Your Needs:

Reflect on the various tips and techniques discussed in this book. Consider which ones resonate with you and align with your lifestyle and preferences.

2. Set Realistic Goals:

Identify specific goals you want to achieve in managing your low back pain. These goals should be realistic, measurable, and time-bound. For example, you might aim to improve your posture, incorporate regular exercise, or reduce pain medication reliance.

3. Prioritise Self-Care:

Self-care is a vital aspect of managing low back pain. Make time for activities that promote relaxation, stress reduction, and overall well-being. Consider incorporating practices like journaling, meditation, or engaging in hobbies you enjoy.

4. Build a Routine:

Establish a daily routine that incorporates the strategies and techniques that work best for you. This routine might include exercises, stretches, relaxation practices, and posture checks. Consistency is key in maintaining long-term benefits.

Self-Care Practices for Sustainable Pain Relief

To ensure your pain management plan is sustainable, it's essential to prioritise self-care. Here are some self-care practices to consider:

1. Journaling:

Keep a pain journal to track your symptoms, triggers, and the effectiveness of various strategies. Journaling can help you identify patterns, track progress, and make informed decisions about your pain management plan.

2. Tracking Progress:

Regularly assess your progress towards your goals. Keep a log of the strategies you've implemented and note any improvements or challenges. Celebrate small victories along the way to stay motivated.

3. Mindfulness and Stress Reduction:

Incorporate mindfulness practices, deep breathing exercises, and stress reduction techniques into your daily routine. These practices can help you stay centered, reduce stress levels, and manage pain more effectively.

4. Seeking Support:

Connect with others who are also managing low back pain. Online communities, support groups, or forums can provide valuable support, empathy, and insights. Share your experiences and learn from others who are on a similar journey.

Resources for Ongoing Support

In your quest for sustainable pain relief, it's essential to have access to ongoing support and additional resources. Here are a few suggestions:

1. Online Communities:

Join online communities or social media groups dedicated to low back pain management. These platforms offer a space to share experiences, ask questions, and receive support from individuals who understand your challenges.

2. Professional Support:

Continue working with qualified spinal therapists, such as chiropractors, physical therapists, or pain specialists. They can provide ongoing guidance, adjustments to your treatment plan, and support as needed.

3. Additional Reading:

Explore books, articles, and reputable websites that provide further information on low back pain management. Educating yourself about the latest research and strategies can empower you to make informed decisions about your health.

4. Supportive Networks:

Lean on your personal support system, including friends, family, and loved ones. Share your journey, communicate your needs, and allow them to offer assistance and encouragement when needed.

Conclusion:

Creating a sustainable plan for managing low back pain involves developing a personalised approach, prioritising self-care, and seeking ongoing support. By incorporating the strategies discussed in this book, such as setting realistic goals, tracking progress, and engaging in self-care practices, you can establish a plan that works for you. Remember to be patient, celebrate progress, and adjust your plan as needed. With the right tools, support, and dedication, you can create a sustainable pain management plan that leads to long-term relief and improved quality of life.

16

Conclusion: Embracing a Holistic Approach to Relieve Low Back Pain

Throughout this book, we have explored various practical tips, strategies, and holistic approaches to relieve low back pain. As we conclude this journey, let's recap the key takeaways and reinforce the importance of adopting a holistic approach to finding long-term relief and improved well-being.

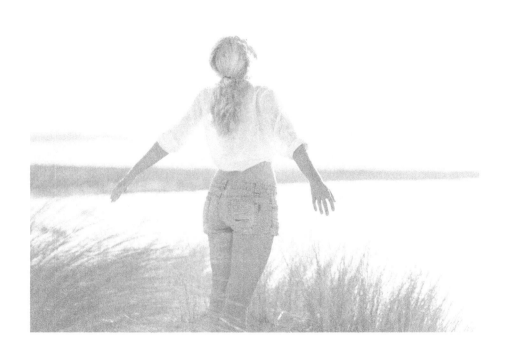

1. Understanding Low Back Pain:

Low back pain can have multiple causes, including muscle strain, poor posture, herniated discs, and emotional factors. It is essential to address the root causes and consider the mind-body connection in our approach to pain management.

2. Creating a Supportive Environment:

Ergonomic work spaces, proper sleep posture, and back-friendly home environments contribute to reduced strain on the back and support a pain-free lifestyle.

3. Gentle Movement and Exercise:

Regular movement and exercises like stretching, yoga, and tai chi promote flexibility, strengthen core muscles, and improve overall back health. It is crucial to exercise with caution, listen to our bodies, and prioritize proper form.

4. Mind-Body Techniques for Pain Relief:

Mindfulness meditation, relaxation techniques, and stress reduction practices play a significant role in managing low back pain. These techniques promote relaxation, reduce stress, and alleviate pain by harnessing the power of the mind-body connection.

5. Nutrition and Lifestyle Choices:

The foods we consume and our lifestyle choices can either contribute to or alleviate inflammation and low back pain. A diet rich in anti-inflammatory foods, maintaining a healthy weight, and proper hydration support a healthy back and overall well-being.

By adopting a holistic approach, we recognise that managing low back pain requires addressing physical, emotional, and lifestyle factors. It is a comprehensive journey that integrates various strategies into our daily lives for long-term relief and improved well-being.

Now, it's time for you, the reader, to take action. Implement the practical tips, strategies, and self-care practices discussed in this book. Develop a personalised plan that encompasses a supportive environment, gentle movement, mindfulness, nutrition, and complementary therapies. Embrace the mindset of self-care and be patient with your progress.

Remember, finding long-term relief from low back pain is not a quick fix but a journey of self-discovery and self-care. Be kind to yourself, celebrate small victories, and adjust your plan as needed. Seek professional guidance, join supportive communities, and engage in ongoing learning.

You have the power to alleviate your low back pain and improve your overall well-being. Embrace the holistic approach and commit to making positive changes in your daily life. With dedication and perseverance, you can find relief, restore your back's health, and live a fulfilling life free from the burden of low back pain.

Wishing you a pain-free and vibrant future!

Peter Bennett

Appendix: Resources for Low Back Pain

Here are some reputable resources available in the United States and the United Kingdom that provide valuable information, support, and resources for managing low back pain. These organizations and websites offer a wealth of knowledge, guidance, and additional tools to help you navigate your low back pain journey.

Please note that the information provided is accurate as of the time of writing this book, but it is always a good idea to verify the current information on the respective websites.

United States:

1. American Chiropractic Association (ACA) – Website: www.acatoday.org

The ACA is the largest professional association in the United States representing chiropractors. Their website offers educational resources, information about low back pain, and a search tool to find chiropractors in your area.

2. National Institute of Neurological Disorders and Stroke (NINDS) – Website: www.ninds.nih.gov

NINDS, part of the National Institutes of Health, provides information and resources on various neurological disorders, including low back pain. Their website offers research updates, treatment options, and tips for managing pain.

4. Mayo Clinic – Website: www.mayoclinic.org

The Mayo Clinic is a renowned medical center that offers comprehensive information on various health conditions, including low back pain. Their website features articles, videos, and self-help tips for managing back pain.

United Kingdom:

1. National Health Service (NHS) – Website: www.nhs.uk

The NHS is the primary healthcare provider in the United Kingdom. Their website offers extensive information on low back pain, including causes, treatment options, and self-care advice.

2. United Chiropractic Association (UCA) - Website: www.unitedchiropractic.org

The UCA is a professional organization representing chiropractors in the UK. Their website provides information on low back pain, advice on choosing a chiropractor, and resources for maintaining a healthy spine.

3. Chartered Society of Physiotherapy (CSP) – Website: www.csp.org.uk

The CSP is a professional organization for physiotherapists in the UK. Their website offers guidance on managing low back pain, exercises, and a search tool to find physiotherapists near you.

4. BackCare – Website: www.backcare.org.uk

BackCare is a UK-based charity dedicated to helping people prevent and manage back pain. Their website provides educational resources, self-help tips, and information on support groups and events.

These resources serve as a starting point for your exploration of low back pain management. They offer reliable information, expert advice, and tools to support your journey toward a healthier, pain-free back. Remember to consult with healthcare professionals and use these resources as supplemental guidance for your specific situation.

Please note that the inclusion of these resources does not imply endorsement or guarantee of their services, and it is always important to verify the information and seek personalised advice from qualified healthcare professionals.

Appendix: About the Author

Dr. Peter Bennett, the author of this book, is a chiropractor and health coach with over 20 years of experience in helping individuals manage and overcome low back pain. With a passion for holistic approaches and a gentle, compassionate style, Dr. Bennett has dedicated his career to improving the health and well-being of his patients.

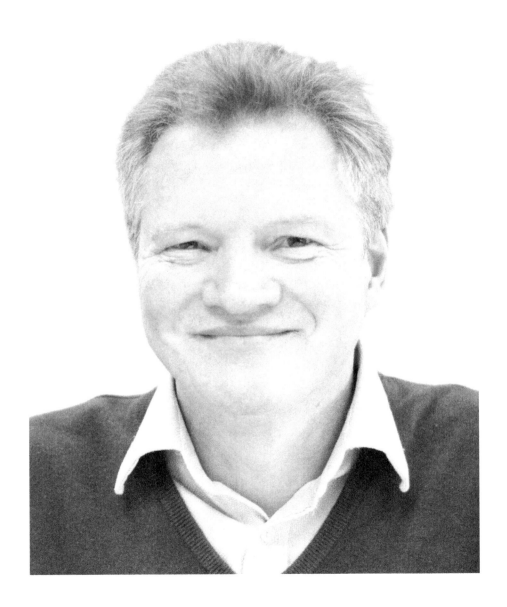

Dr. Bennett completed his chiropractic education at the McTimoney College of Chiropractic, where he gained a deep understanding of the musculoskeletal system and its relationship to overall health. Through his years of practice, he has honed his skills in diagnosing and treating conditions that affect the low back, such as muscle strain, herniated discs, and poor posture.

Beyond his chiropractic expertise, Dr. Bennett is also a health coach. This additional training allows him to take a comprehensive approach to his patients' well-being, considering not only the physical aspects of their health but also their mental, emotional, and lifestyle factors. Dr. Bennett understands that true healing encompasses the whole person, and he is dedicated to supporting his patients on their journey to optimal health.

In addition to his clinical work, Dr. Bennett is a passionate educator. He believes in empowering individuals with knowledge and practical tools to manage their own health. Through workshops, seminars, and public speaking engagements, he shares his expertise and inspires others to take an active role in their well-being.

Dr. Bennett's writing style reflects his commitment to making complex health information accessible and easy to understand. In this book, he presents practical tips, strategies, and insights in an approachable manner, allowing readers to navigate the world of low back pain with clarity and confidence.

While Dr. Bennett's experience and expertise are invaluable, it's important to note that the information provided in this book is not a substitute for personalised medical advice. Each individual's situation is unique, and readers are encouraged to consult with qualified healthcare professionals for guidance tailored to their specific needs.

Dr. Bennett's mission is to empower individuals to take control of their health, find relief from low back pain, and achieve overall well-being. Through his compassionate approach, extensive knowledge, and dedication to his patients, he continues to make a positive impact in the lives of those seeking relief from low back pain.

Please note that the information provided in this appendix is accurate as of the time of writing this book. For the most up-to-date information on Dr. Peter Bennett's work and offerings, please visit his official website www.yourspinalhealth.com.

Printed in Great Britain
by Amazon

24705747R00056